D0296883

SUPER FOOD

COCONUT

B L O O M S B U R Y

LONDON · OXFORD · NEW YORK · NEW DELHI · SYDNEY

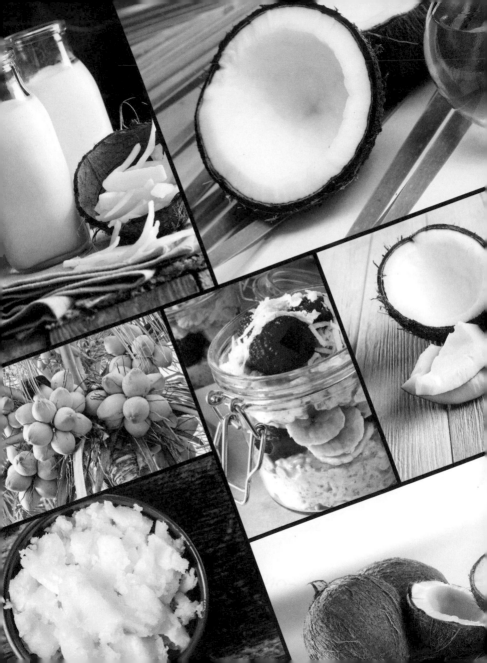

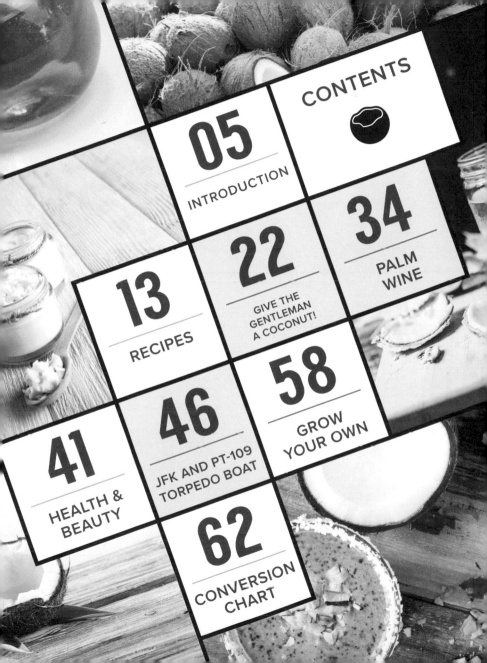

CONTENTS

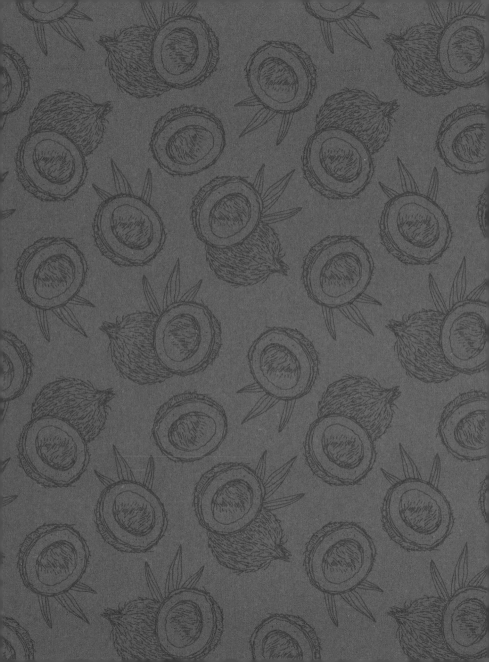

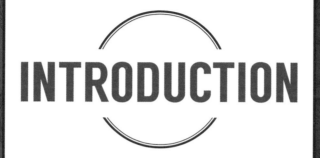

INTRODUCTION

'The Cocoa Nut is, of all
Palms, most deservedly
valued as one of the
greatest of the many
blessings showered down
by a bountiful Providence
upon the inhabitants
of a tropical clime.'

Thomas Treloar,
The Prince of Palms, 1852

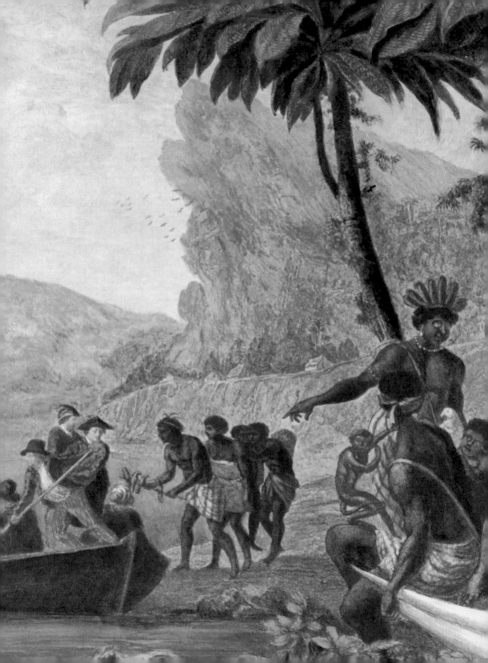

HISTORY

The earliest references to the coconut (*cocos nucifera L.*) are in ancient Sanskrit texts, where it is referred to as *kalpavriksha*, meaning 'tree which gives everything you need', showing the coconut's many uses were recognised and appreciated from early times. It is still revered in Indian religion and used in Hindu ceremonies, representing good luck and prosperity.

The coconut appears to have originated in the islands of the south Pacific, from where it spread to southern India, although its distribution route and indeed its origin are debated. A recent study has examined the DNA of coconuts and identified two distinct types, one found in the Pacific basin between Asia and America and the other in the Indo-Atlantic basin between Asia and the Caribbean via Western

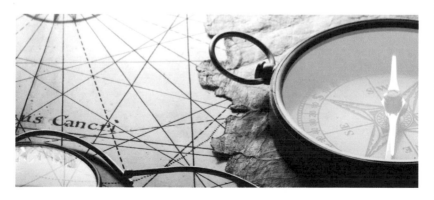

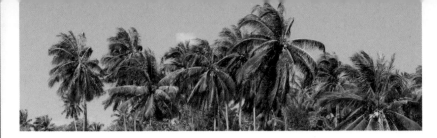

Africa, which suggests that the coconut was first cultivated in Asia and spread both east and west from there.

It is likely that the coconut was carried to other lands by seafarers plying their way along ancient trade routes. In the account of Sinbad's 5th voyage (based on the adventures of Eastern traders in the 8th–9th centuries) Sinbad describes how he was shown a method of harvesting coconuts by throwing stones at the apes in the palm trees 'the apes out of revenge threw cocoa-nuts at us fast ... by this stratagem we filled our bags with cocoa-nuts'. Sinbad was collecting these coconuts to trade in exchange for pepper with the nearby island.

It is possible, however, that the coconut, with its light waterproof shell, could have spread independently by floating across the sea until it reached another shore and rooted itself. By whatever means, by the 6th century AD the coconut is thought to have arrived in Egypt from India, and by medieval times trading routes had bought it as far as western Europe. The exotic coconut was such a rarity that it was used as an art material by jewellers who removed the outer husks, polished the shell until it was smooth and decorated it with precious gems. A beautiful example of a coconut cup can be seen in the Ashmolean museum in Oxford. These cups were signs of status in wealthy families and were passed down the generations.

The coconut was becoming more widespread. Marco Polo, the Venetian explorer, was familiar with the coconut when he encountered it on his travels in Sumatra in 1210, referring to it as *nux indica* (the Indian nut). He writes that 'the cavity of this pulp is filled with a liquor clear as water, cool, and better flavoured and more delicate than wine or any other kind of drink whatever'.

> *It is generally accepted that the coconut first got its modern name from Portuguese explorers in the 16th century.*

In March 1521 the Italian explorer Ludivico di Varthema visited India and wrote about the 'tenga tree' (the Malayalim name for the coconut) which he called 'the most fruitful tree in the world': 'Ten useful things are derived from this tree. The first utility is wood to burn; nuts to eat; ropes for maritime navigation; thin stuffs which, when they are dyed, appear to be made of silk; charcoal in the greatest perfection; wine; water; oil and sugar; and with its leaves which fall, that is when a branch falls, they cover the houses ... Were I to declare to you in what manner it accomplishes so many things you would not believe it, neither could you understand it.'

It is generally accepted that the coconut first got its modern name from Portuguese explorers in

the 16th century. They called the fruit 'coco', which means 'head', because the shell looks like a face with its three holes suggesting eyes and mouth. Subsequently the fruit became known as the coco nut. It is probable that the Portuguese and Spanish explorers took the coconut to the New World with them, although it was still rare in the 19th century, as an American missionary, writing from Ceylon (Sri Lanka) notes that he will make some remarks '... about [the palmyra tree and] the cocoa-nut tree, neither of which I believe is in the United States'.

By the end of the 19th century, the mighty British empire was transporting goods around the world, and the coconut now became a familiar sight, initially as an exotic fruit to eat, and then, as it became more common, in manufacturing. The by-products were used in a variety of industries, for example the manufacture of coir matting, which achieved fame when it was used as a floor covering at St George's Chapel, Windsor, at the christening of the future King Edward VII in 1842.

HEALTH BENEFITS

Regarded for centuries as an essential foodstuff in tropical countries, the coconut was for years not considered particularly healthy due to the levels of saturated fat it contains. Coconuts do contain a significant amount of fat, but the fats are what are known as medium-chain triglycerides (MCTs), which are converted into energy quickly rather than being stored as fat.

This energy boost, which helps with physical performance, is similar to that given by carbohydrates, but without the weight gain and insulin-spike which can lead to health problems, especially in diabetics. Studies have also shown that eating coconut can increase thyroid activity, which helps with stabilising weight and boosts the immune system.

MCTs also help boost the body's ketone levels which help maintain good brain health and avoid neurological problems such as dementia. Around half the fat in the coconut is a fat called lauric acid which is converted by the body into an antibacterial and antiviral compound called monolaurin which strengthens immunity and fights infection and viruses. Lauric acid does raise bad cholesterol levels but to a greater degree it boosts good cholesterols which prevent blood vessels becoming blocked, thus countering the risk of heart disease. It is advised to eat coconuts in moderation though, due to this high fat content.

Coconuts are also full of vitamins including Vitamin C, essential for boosting the immune system, and Vitamin E, which is needed to promote new cell development and helps maintain good skin health. They also contain the B vitamins B1,

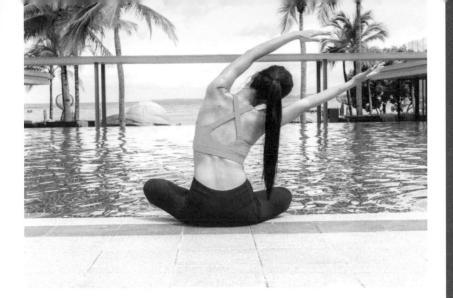

B3, B5 and B6, which work together to release energy from food and keep the nervous system, blood cells and skin healthy.

Coconuts are also rich in minerals including iron, potassium, calcium, selenium and zinc, all essential to good health. Potassium helps fight depression and regulates heart rate as well as being good for digestion. Calcium is good for bone health, while zinc and selenium help repair cells and fight infection. Iron is an essential mineral as it aids the production of red blood cells which carry oxygen round the body.

Coconut water is high in electrolytes which are essential for hydration, digestion and a good metabolism. It contains cytokinins which fight ageing, cancer, and thrombosis.

Coconuts contain folates which prevent stroke and heart disease, as well as guarding against birth defects in unborn babies. They are rich in fibre so help you stay fuller for longer and thus avoid overeating.

It is not surprising that for centuries the coconut has been regarded as a unique source of all the nutrition a man needs to survive!

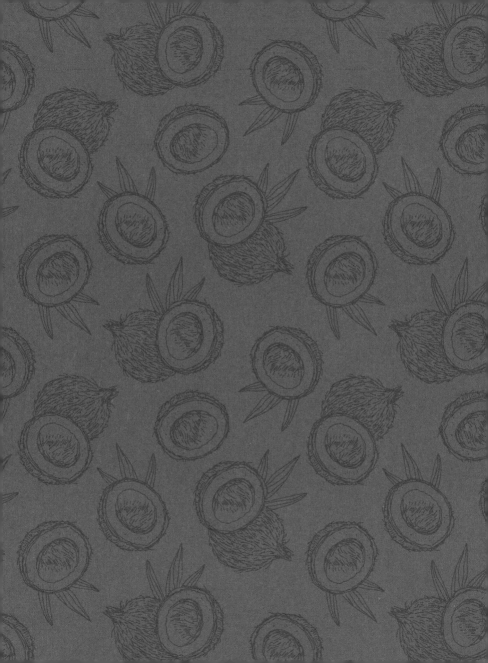

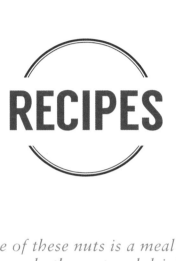

RECIPES

'*One of these nuts is a meal for a man, both meat and drink.*'

The travels of Marco Polo
(1254–1324)

SERVES: 2
PREPARATION: 5 MINUTES

BREAKFAST
SMOOTHIES

The creamy taste of coconut is ideal for making delicious and healthy dairy-free smoothies to give you a taste of the tropics.

INGREDIENTS

- 200ml coconut milk
- 1 banana
- a few mango chunks (you can use frozen ones)
- ¼ melon, cut into chunks
- juice of ½ lime
- 1 tsp dessicated coconut

MANGO, BANANA & MELON

Bananas contain potassium which is great for mood, and mango is rich in Vitamin C to boost your immune system. Place all the ingredients in a blender and whizz until completely smooth.

INGREDIENTS

- 200ml coconut water
- a handful of spinach leaves
- 100g mixed berries (you can use frozen ones)
- 1 pear, peeled and cored

COCONUT WATER, SPINACH & BERRIES

Coconut water contains electrolytes which are great for maintaining good heart health and hydration, while berries are high in antioxidants and spinach is rich in folic acid. A super-smoothie! Blend the ingredients as above.

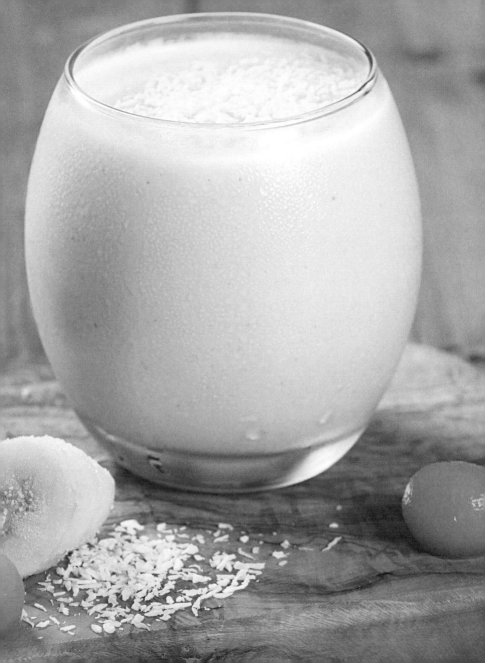

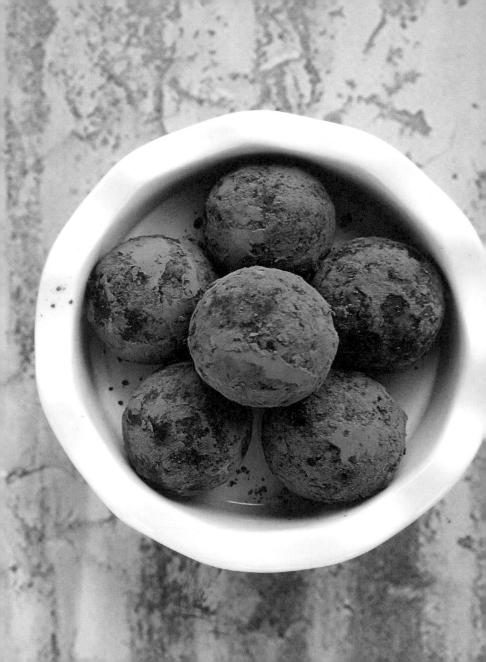

MAKES: 12 BALLS
PREPARATION: 10 MINUTES

ENERGY BALLS

These quick and easy no-cook balls of goodness are packed with nutrients and make a perfect healthy snack.

INGREDIENTS

- 100g dates, chopped
- 50g chopped walnuts
- 1 tsp cocoa powder, plus extra for dusting
- 1 tbsp cashew nut butter
- 20ml orange juice
- 20ml dessicated coconut

METHOD

Place all the ingredients in a blender and whizz until fully combined. Shake a thin layer of cocoa powder onto a plate. Form 12 balls from the mixture with your hands and roll them around in the cocoa powder until lightly dusted. Refrigerate.

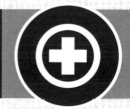

COCONUT WATER WAS USED IN THE SECOND WORLD WAR IN PLACE OF SALINE WHEN NONE WAS AVAILABLE. DUE TO THE FACT THAT IT IS USUALLY STERILE.

SERVES: 2
PREPARATION: 10 MINUTES
COOKING TIME: 4 MINUTES

💡 TOP TIP

If you prefer you can substitute the garlic mayonnaise with a Thai sweet chilli dip.

INGREDIENTS

For the prawns:

- 3 tbsp plain flour
- 1 egg, beaten
- 6 tbsp desiccated coconut
- 6 tbsp panko breadcrumbs
- 1 tbsp vegetable oil
- 10 large prawns with tails intact

For the dip:

- 3 tbsp mayonnaise
- 1 clove garlic, crushed
- 1 tbsp lemon juice

COCONUT
PRAWNS

These quick and easy prawns make a delicious starter or snack. The coconut adds an extra texture to the crispy coating.

METHOD

Place the flour in one dish, the beaten egg in a second dish, and the coconut and breadcrumbs, mixed together, in a third dish.

Heat the oil. Dip the prawns in the flour, then shake off any excess flour and dip them in the egg. Finally roll the prawns around in the coconut mix, making sure they are coated evenly, before frying them in the oil for a couple of minutes on each side.

Mix together the dip ingredients and serve on the side.

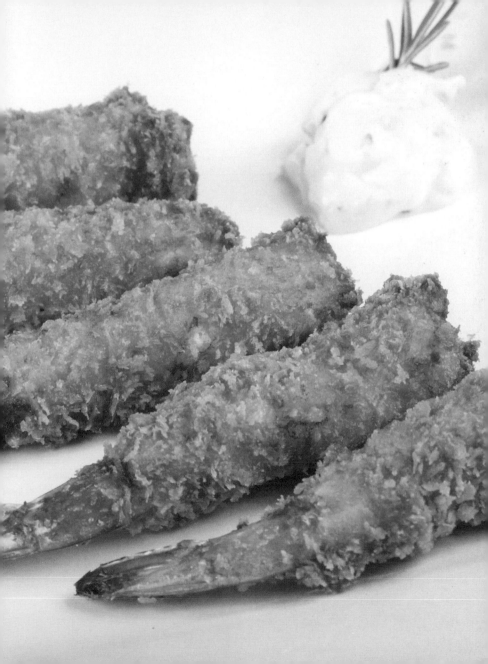

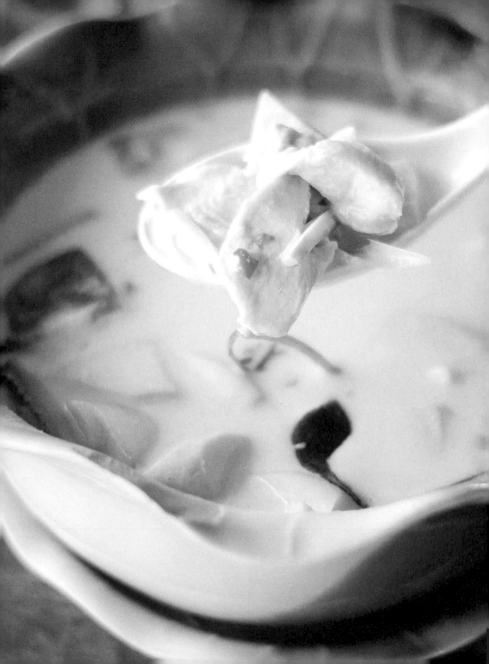

SERVES: 4
PREPARATION: 10 MINUTES
COOKING TIME: 20 MINUTES

INGREDIENTS

- 1 small onion
- a thumb-sized piece of ginger
- 1 red pepper
- 1 tbsp vegetable oil
- stick of lemongrass
- 3 kaffir lime leaves
- ½ jar of red curry paste
- 100g shitake or oyster mushrooms
- 2 chicken breasts
- 200ml chicken stock
- 400ml can coconut milk
- 1 tsp fish sauce
- 1 tsp sugar
- juice of 1 lime
- a bunch of fresh coriander
- salt and freshly ground black pepper

THAI COCONUT CHICKEN SOUP

Smooth coconut milk and calming chicken balance the spicy Thai flavours of lemongrass, ginger and lime in this deliciously comforting soup.

METHOD

Finely chop the onion and ginger, and slice the red pepper thinly. Heat the oil gently in a saucepan and add the onion with the ginger, lemongrass, lime leaves and curry paste. Stir frequently while cooking until the onion is translucent, then add the pepper and mushrooms and stir for another minute.

Chop the chicken breasts and add to the pan, together with the chicken stock, coconut milk, fish sauce and sugar. Simmer for 20 minutes. Remove the chicken breasts, shred into small pieces and return to the saucepan.

Finally add the lime juice and most of the coriander, reserving a few for the garnish, and season to taste.

Garnish with the remaining coriander leaves and serve immediately.

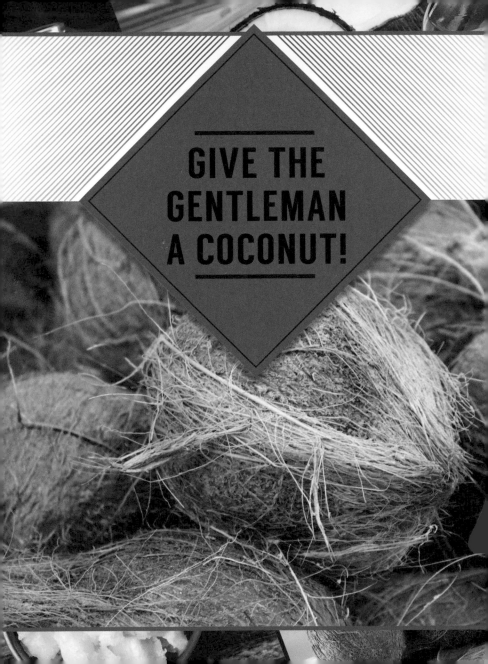

GIVE THE GENTLEMAN A COCONUT!

Throwing objects at targets for fun has long been a standard pastime at a day out at the fair.

Early precursors of the coconut shy (the use of the word 'shy' as a word for 'throw' dates to the 18th century) include games such as Knock-em-down, and a game of uncertain origin called Aunt Sally, where an effigy was pelted with balls or sticks ('sally' means to pitch forward).

Aunt Sally may have evolved from a far less pleasant game played on Shrove Tuesday called 'cock-throwing' where people threw weighted sticks at a live cock. This was outlawed in the 18th century after being condemned by figures such as the satirist William Hogarth who observed the practice of '... throwing at a cock, – an ordinary amusement at Shrovetime, which all the vigilance of the police has hitherto been ineffectual in removing' (*The First Stage of Cruelty*, 1812). This game fortunately evolved into a more benign form where the 'cock' became a target made of lead cast in moulds representing birds, men, horses and other devices which were set up and 'shyed at with dumps from a small distance agreed upon by the parties'.

So how did the coconut end up being the target of choice?

> *For the sum of a penny, you could have three throws with sticks 'with the prospect of getting a cocoa nut'.*

In Kingston-upon-Thames, Surrey, there is a pub called 'The Cocoanut' (the original spelling) which provides a possible clue. There were once several mills on the Hogsmill river near the pub which were involved in the coconut industry, the main one being Middle Mill which manufactured coconut nut fibre, making such products as coir mats. The other two mills may also have dealt with the by-products of this industry. It has been suggested that the first occurrence of a coconut shy was at the annual Pleasure Fair held in Kingston in 1867, when the local paper reported that for the sum of a penny, you could have three throws with sticks 'with the prospect of getting a cocoa nut' or some other prize. It seems likely that the coconuts originated from the mills.

Certainly from the late 19th century the coconut shy became a common sight at fairs around the country. Coconuts would originally have been an exotic prize to win, although they soon became common, as it was noted that 'in nearly every country fair, and in almost all the open spaces round London at holiday seasons, the cocoa-nut plays so conspicuous a part that every child is acquainted with it ... .' The term 'coconut shy' first appeared in the dictionary at the turn of the 20th century, the sticks were replaced by wooden balls, and now the coconut shy is firmly established as a traditional part of fairground entertainment.

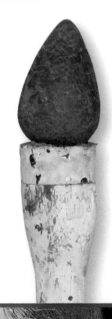

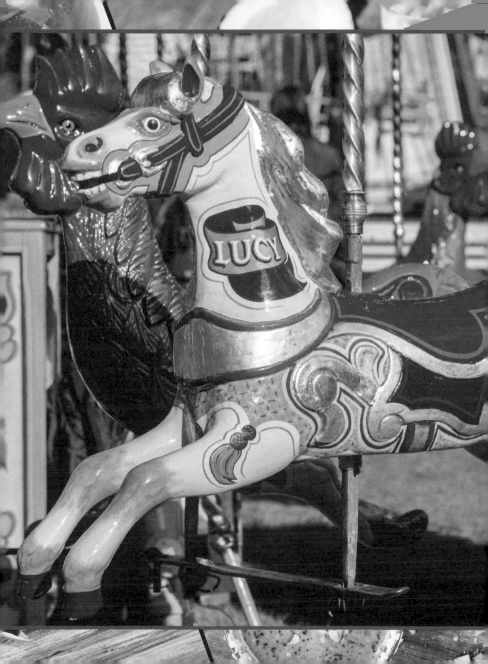

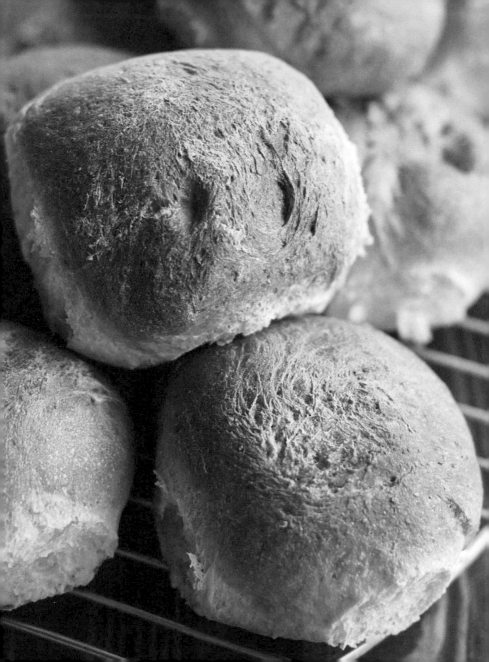

PAN DE COCO

MAKES: 12 ROLLS
PREPARATION: 1 HOUR
COOKING TIME: 20-25 MINUTES

 TOP TIP

For a shiny glaze, brush the top of the rolls with beaten egg before baking.

INGREDIENTS

- 2 tbsp soft brown sugar
- 2 tsp dried yeast granules
- 60ml warm water
- 475g plain flour
- 3/4 tsp salt
- 2 eggs, beaten well
- 250ml coconut milk
- 40g butter, melted

Pan de coco or 'coconut bread' is a popular bread from the Philippines. The recipe probably originated in Honduras and was bought to the Philippines by the Spanish during the 16th or 17th century. It is usually served while still warm as a breakfast or afternoon snack with coffee or hot chocolate.

METHOD

Place the dessicated coconut, brown sugar, yeast and water into a bowl and stir well. Leave in a warm place for half an hour, or until the yeast has become bubbly. Sift the flour and salt into a large bowl, and add the yeast mixture, beaten eggs, coconut milk and melted butter. Mix the ingredients together until fully combined.

Turn the dough out onto a floured board and knead for five minutes until soft and elastic. Cover with a clean tea towel and leave to rise until doubled in size.

Knock back the dough and divide into 12 rolls. Place on a greased baking tray, cover with the tea towel and leave to rise again. Preheat oven to 180°C/350°F/gas mark 4.

Bake the rolls for 20–25 minutes or until golden brown.

FISH CURRY

INGREDIENTS

For the curry paste:

- 1 green chilli
- 1 garlic clove
- a thumb-sized piece of ginger
- 1 tsp ground cumin
- 1 tsp ground turmeric
- juice of ½ lime
- a handful of coriander leaves

For the curry:

- 2 tbsp vegetable oil
- 1 onion
- 500g cod, diced
- 1 sweet potato
- 400ml tin coconut milk
- 200g green beans
- salt
- a handful of coriander leaves
- 1 lime

This classic Asian dish provides you with the low-fat protein of fish spiced up with the clean refreshing flavours of coriander, lime and chilli, with the coconut milk blending it all together.

METHOD

Chop and blend together all the curry paste ingredients, adding water if needed to create a smooth paste.

Heat the oil and gently fry the paste for a couple of minutes, stirring frequently. Finely chop the onion and cook on a low heat until it is translucent, before adding the fish and the sweet potato, peeled and diced.

Stir for a further couple of minutes and then pour in the coconut milk and add the beans. Simmer for a further ten minutes until the beans and potatoes are soft. Add salt to taste. Garnish with the coriander leaves and serve with wedges of lime.

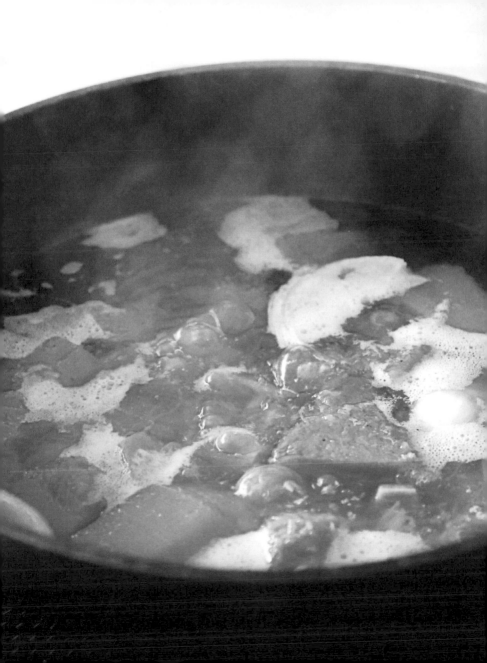

MANGO & COCONUT SALAD

SERVES: 2
PREPARATION: 15 MINUTES

  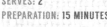

DF GF VG V

A tropical pairing of smooth mango and crunchy toasted coconut flakes makes this beautiful little salad — a lovely side dish to accompany grilled fish or chicken.

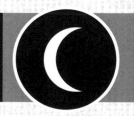

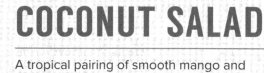

IN 1985 THE MALDIVES ADOPTED THE COCONUT PALM AS THEIR NATIONAL TREE — IT FEATURES ON THE NATIONAL EMBLEM AND SYMBOLISES LIVELIHOOD AND PROSPERITY.

INGREDIENTS

- 2 tbsp unsweetened coconut flakes
- 1 tbsp extra virgin olive oil
- 2 tsp soft brown sugar
- zest and juice of ½ lime
- salt and freshly ground black pepper
- 1 ripe mango, peeled and sliced
- 1 red pepper, sliced thinly
- 200g baby leaf salad

METHOD

Heat a small frying pan and gently toss the flaked coconut in the pan until tinged golden brown. Leave to cool.

Mix together the olive oil, sugar, lime zest and lime juice in a small bowl. Season to taste.

Place the mango and red peppers in a serving bowl and pour the dressing over, tossing the ingredients together to ensure they are thoroughly coated.

Serve on a bed of salad leaves with the toasted coconut scattered on top.

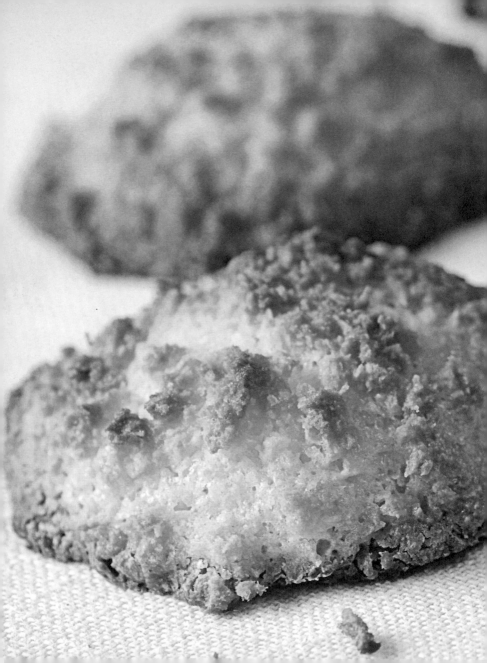

COCONUT
PYRAMIDS

The traditional taste of childhood, coconut pyramids have been a popular party food for decades and are easy to make.

INGREDIENTS

- 2 egg whites
- 80g icing sugar
- 2 tbsp almond flour
- 170g dessicated coconut
- ½ tsp vanilla essence

METHOD

Preheat oven to 160°C/325°F/gas mark 3.

Whisk the egg whites until stiff. Sift in the icing sugar and add the flour, dessicated coconut and vanilla essence.

Divide the mixture into 12 pyramid shapes and place on a greased baking tray. Bake for 10–12 minutes or until light brown in colour.

Allow your pyramids to cool fully as they will harden in the process.

IN *THE STORY OF THE TREASURE SEEKERS* BY E. NESBIT (1899), ONE OF THE CHILDREN'S MOST TREASURED POSSESSIONS IS 'TWO-PENNYWORTH OF COCONUT CANDY'.

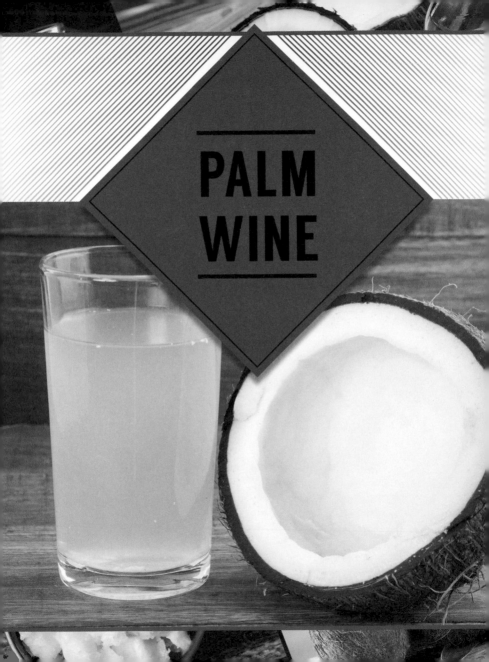

PALM WINE

> '**Palmwine, palmwine, palmwine, palmwine!**
>
> **Let's all drink palmwine with all our might!**'
>
> **Amos Tutuola, *The Palm-Wine Drunkard* (1952)**

Palm wine is an alcoholic drink made from the fermented sap of the palm tree and enjoyed by millions of people across the Carribbean, Africa, Asia and South America. It is known by many names, including *kachae* (Thailand), *malafu* (Congo), *poyo* (Sierra Leone) and *Tuk tnout choo* (Cambodia). Palm wine is an important part of daily life and is used in ceremonies such as weddings and other special occasions.

The sap is extracted by a palm wine tapper who drills a hole into the trunk of the tree and collects the liquid, which is sweet and non-alcoholic at this point. The sap immediately begins to ferment, however, due to naturally occurring yeasts, and is ready to drink after about two hours, by which time its alcoholic content is around 4%. It is usually drunk within 24 hours, after which time the liquid becomes vinegary. Palm wine is a cloudy white colour and tastes sweet.

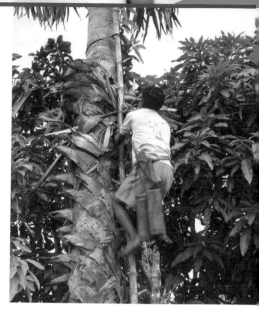

It is not only humans who enjoy the wine – recently chimpanzees in Guinea have been observed seeking out the by-products of the palm wine industry such as wine-soaked leaves and enjoying an alcoholic tipple!

Palm wine can also be distilled, traditionally by heating in earthenware stills, to produce an extremely potent alcohol, sometimes compared to whisky or rum, and with an alcoholic content of around 50%! This also has different names – it is known as *arak* in South Asia and *feni* in India.

ICE CREAM

Coconut milk is here sweetened with maple syrup and vanilla for a beautifully rich and flavoursome ice cream.

INGREDIENTS

- 6 egg yolks
- 400ml tin coconut milk
- 350ml single cream
- 250ml maple syrup
- 1 tsp vanilla essence
- 60g desiccated coconut

To serve:

- chocolate sauce
- a handful of peanuts

METHOD

Whisk the egg yolks and gradually add the coconut milk, single cream, maple syrup and vanilla essence. Finally add the dessicated coconut.

If you are using an ice-cream machine chill the mixture for a couple of hours before freezing according to the machine instructions. If not then freeze for a couple of hours, break up the chunks and whisk again. Repeat a couple more times over the next few hours, then freeze again until fully set.

Serve with the chocolate sauce and peanuts scattered on top.

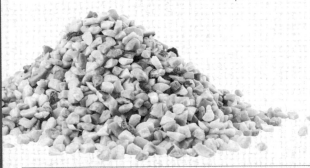

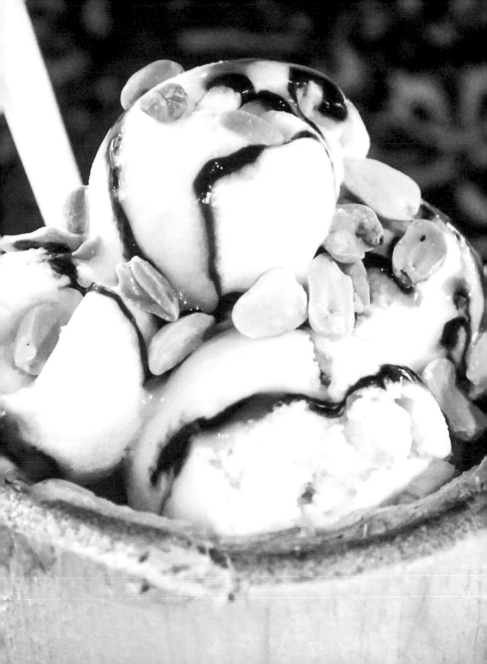

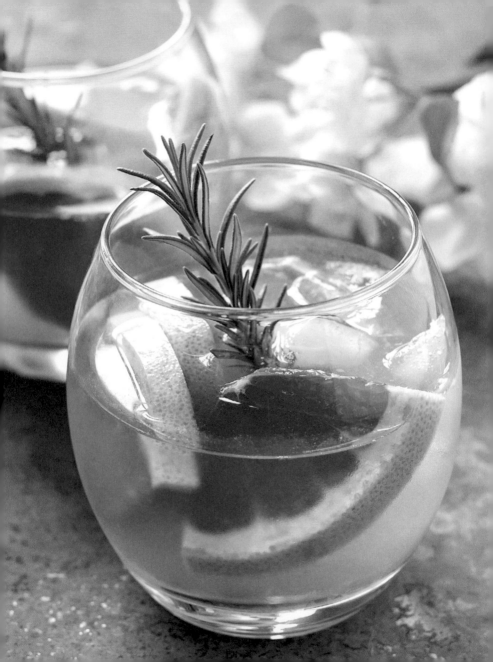

SERVES: 2
PREPARATION: **5 MINUTES**

VODKA & GRAPEFRUIT COCKTAIL

Coconut water has a naturally sweet flavour which offsets the tangy grapefruit in this classy variation on the classic vodka and orange.

INGREDIENTS

- a handful of ice cubes
- 50ml coconut water
- 20ml vodka
- 20ml pink grapefruit juice (approx ¼ squeezed fruit)

METHOD

Mix together and serve over ice with a slice of grapefruit.

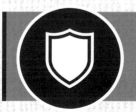

THE GILBERT ISLANDERS OF KIRIBATI TRADITIONALLY WORE ARMOUR WOVEN FROM COCONUT HUSK ROPE TO PROTECT THEMSELVES FROM THEIR ENEMIES.

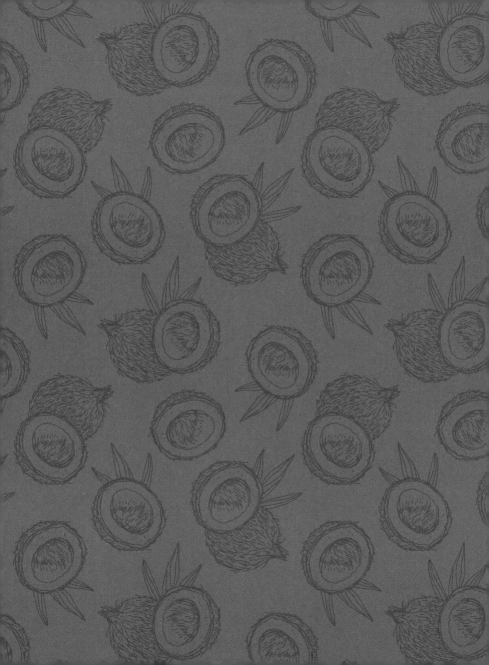

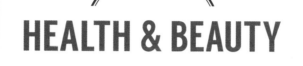

HEALTH & BEAUTY

*'They are immoderately fond of
cocoa-nut oil ... a great quantity
of which they not only pour
upon their head and shoulders,
but rub the body all over,
briskly, with a smaller quantity.
And none but those who have
seen this practice, can easily
conceive how the appearance of
the skin is improved by it.'*

From Vol 1 of Captain Cook's last
voyage to the Pacific Ocean in the
years 1776, 1777, 1778, 1780.

HONEY, LEMON & COCONUT OIL BRIGHTENING MASK

Coconut oil's small molecular structure allows it to penetrate skin pores to soften rough skin from within. Honey is a natural humectant, which hydrates skin cells, while fresh lemon juice is a natural astringent, which helps tighten and shrink large pores.

INGREDIENTS

- 1 tbsp organic coconut oil
- 2 tsp Manuka honey
- ½ tsp lemon juice

 TOP TIP

Use organic coconut oil where possible so that you can avoid skin irritations. Processed coconut oils can sometimes contain additives that may cause allergic reactions.

METHOD

Combine the ingredients in a bowl. On clean, damp skin, preferably after a gentle exfoliation, apply a generous layer of the mask. A bath is a great place for a face mask as the steam from the warm water helps the skin to absorb the nutrients.

Relax for ten minutes. Rinse the mask off thoroughly with clean, warm water. Pat dry with a soft towel to reveal fresher, softer skin.

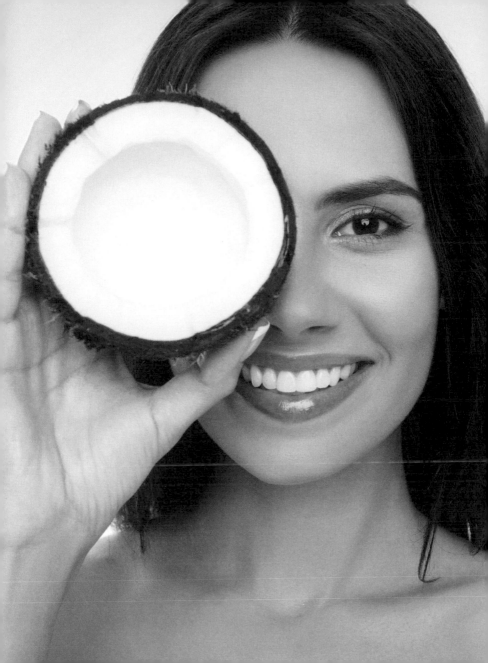

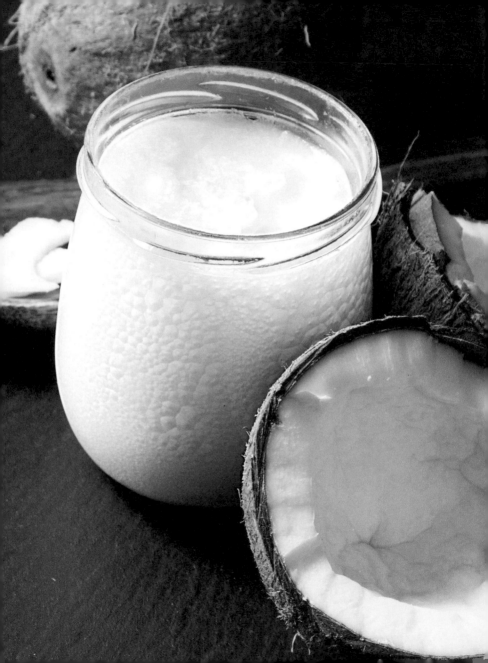

NATURAL MOISTURISER

Coconut oil's luxurious creamy texture makes it the perfect 100% natural moisturiser for face and body.

After you shower or bathe, apply coconut oil directly onto your warm, damp skin and allow the natural oils to be absorbed by gently massaging in.

Your skin will feel smooth and nourished, and you can relax in the knowledge that you have used a totally natural product with no harmful chemicals.

TOP TIP

You could also add in a few drops of your favourite essential oil to give your skin, and senses, an extra treat!

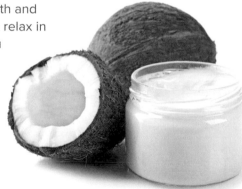

 **COCONUTS CONTAIN VITAMIN E WHICH IS NEEDED TO PROMOTE NEW CELL DEVELOPMENT.**

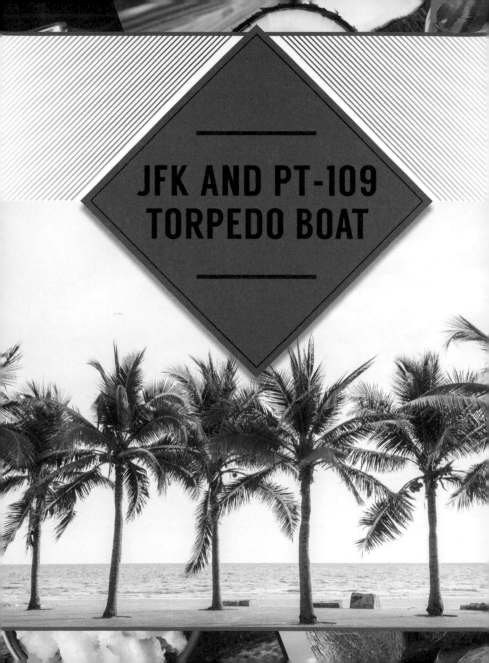

JFK AND PT-109
TORPEDO BOAT

During the Second World War, future US president John F. Kennedy served in the US navy, and was posted to the newly formed PT (Patrol Torpedo) Squadron, which had been based in the South Pacific since 1941.

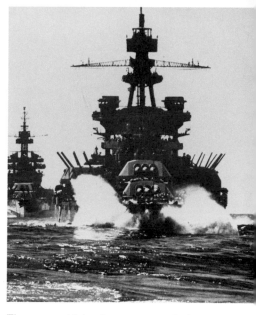

In 1943 the now-promoted Lieutenant Kennedy was given the command of Motor Torpedo Boat PT-109. On August 2nd the navy dispatched a fleet of PT boats, including PT-109, to intercept a Japanese convoy which was delivering supplies to enemy troops in the Solomon islands. PT-109 had a problem with its radar and the crew were unaware of the approach of a Japanese destroyer, the *Amagiri*, until it was right upon them and crashed through their boat. PT-109 was critically damaged and caught fire.

Things were bleak; two of the crew had been killed and one had been seriously burned in the fire. Kennedy managed to rally the survivors in the water and get them to climb onto the remains of the wrecked boat. By the next day though it was clear they had to abandon the sinking PT-109.

The nearest islands were occupied by Japanese troops, so Kennedy decided to aim for a small island which was three miles away. The only way was to swim, and Kennedy pulled the wounded crewmember the whole way, towing him by the strap of his life jacket with his teeth.

The exhausted crew of PT-109 crawled onto the island known as Plum Pudding island and hid among the trees. The relief of being out of the sea was short-lived however as there was no fresh water and nothing to eat. After two days they had to swim to a nearby island where they found coconuts to give them some nourishment, but after a further few days they were becoming sick and despondent. Kennedy tried to swim out into the channel to see if he could get help but without success.

> *Kennedy picked up a fallen coconut shell and scratched a message inside it …*

Finally Kennedy and another man swam to the island of Nauru and found some supplies. They also spotted some native islanders, with whom they made contact the next day. Kennedy picked up a fallen coconut shell and scratched inside it the following message:

NAURU ISL.   COMMANDER
NATIVE KNOWS POS'IT
HE CAN PILOT   11 ALIVE
NEED SMALL BOAT   KENNEDY

Kennedy repeated the word 'Rendova' several times, hoping that the men would understand that he wanted them to take the crude message to the PT base there. The scouts, who were called Biuku Gasa and Eroni Kumana, took the coconut shell together with a knife so they could scratch the message out if caught by the Japanese, and paddled off in their canoe.

The next day four natives returned and one walked up to Kennedy, saying, in perfect English, 'I have a message for you, sir'. The message asked Kennedy to return with the natives, and confirmed that the British Navy would 'be in radio communication with the authorities at Rendova, [to] … finalise plans to collect balance of your party'.

That night the rescue arrived in the form of a US PT boat, and Kennedy heard American voices calling to him out of the darkness offering him food. Kennedy responded, with feeling, 'No thanks, I just had a coconut'.

Kennedy received the Navy and Marine Corps medal and the Purple Heart for his heroism. He refused the chance to go home and stayed on the patrol boats. Kennedy kept the coconut shell and it was turned into a paperweight which he kept on his desk at the White House. It is now kept in the John F. Kennedy Presidential Library and Museum.

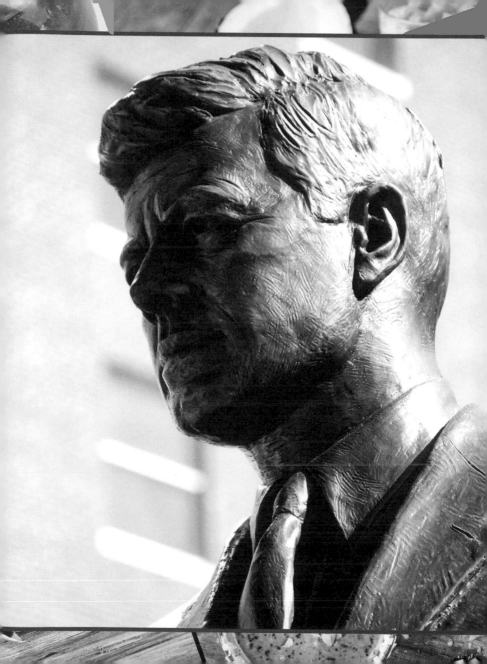

BODY SCRUB

Coconut oil makes a great base for a body scrub as its moisturising properties keep working long after the scrub is washed off for beautifully soft, glowing skin.

METHOD

Mix the sea salt or sugar with the coconut oil. Add a few drops of essential oil like tea tree or lavender for an extra-sensory experience.

In a warm shower or bath, using circular motions, working from your feet upwards to increase your skin's circulation, scrub the skin all over paying particular attention to rougher areas such as elbows and feet.

Rinse off and enjoy the feeling of smooth clean skin.

INGREDIENTS

- 6 tbsp sea salt or brown sugar
- 6 tbsp coconut oil
- few drops essential oil of your choice

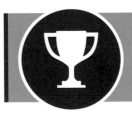

IN 2009 IN KERALA, INDIA, DESIGNERS COMPETED IN VAIN TO REPLACE A LACK OF COCONUT-PICKERS BY INVENTING A MECHANICAL PICKING DEVICE.

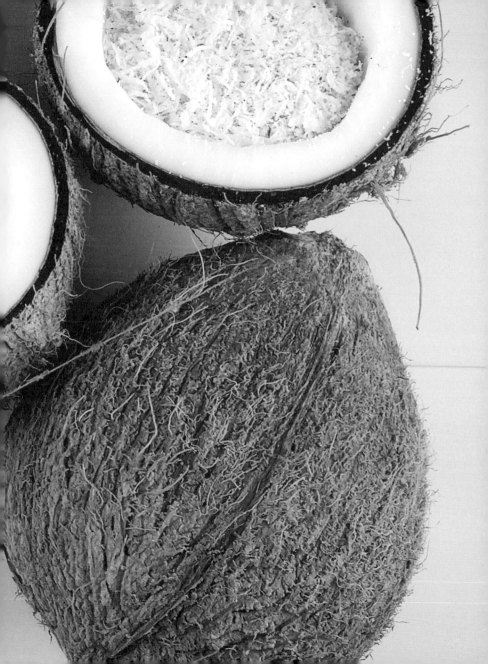

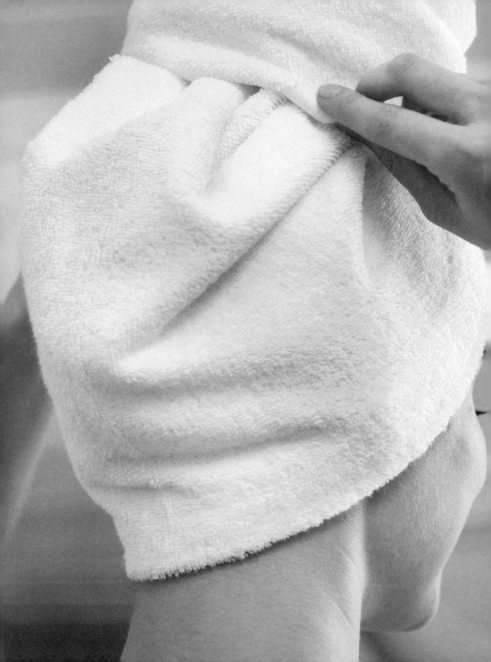

HAIR

Coconut oil is wonderful for hair and is used in countless products. Used in its raw form it can have powerful results, and there are numerous ways it can be applied to achieve beautiful, healthy hair. It also avoids using any harmful chemicals, which may be found in some commercial products.

COCONUT OIL HAIR TOP FIVE

DEEP CONDITIONER – Apply a generous amount of melted coconut oil to clean, damp hair until the hair is completely coated. Wrap your hair in clingfilm around the head and leave for 30 minutes. Rinse well.

SPLIT ENDS REPAIR – Rub a pea-sized amount of coconut oil between flat palms of the hands until the oil is soft. Gently and evenly run your fingers through the ends of clean damp hair before drying, to smooth any frizz and split ends.

DAILY DETANGLE – Rub a pea-sized amount of oil between flat palms of the hands until the oil is soft. Gently and evenly run fingers though your hair from root to tip before combing though with a wide tooth comb.

DANDRUFF REMEDY – Before bed, simply apply melted coconut oil to the scalp and massage well for a few minutes before covering the hair with a towel or clingfilm and leaving on overnight. Wash and rinse well in the morning.

STRENGTH AND GROWTH BOOST – Before bed, massage coconut oil into the scalp and then through the length of your hair to the tips. Leave the treatment on overnight (cover with a towel) and wash thoroughly in the morning for beautifully shiny, sweet-smelling, strong hair.

BEAUTY

Coconut oil makes a useful addition to your beauty kit and it's a great idea to keep a small pot in your beauty bag.

OIL ON

Apply as a luxurious lip balm, or a skin smoother on any dry patches before applying makeup. You can even use it for highlighting with a touch of coconut oil on the high points of your face such as cheekbones, cupid's bow, and brow bones to reflect the light.

OIL OFF

Coconut oil makes a wonderfully gentle eye makeup remover. The oil is smooth and gentle and will nourish the eye area and strengthen your lashes, making this the ideal multi-tasking eye makeup remover, even on hard-to-remove mascara.

Simply rub a pea-sized amount of oil between your hands and massage over closed eyes for a few moments to 'melt' the makeup around your eyes. Pay particular attention to your lashes for maximum moisturizing penetration.

Then using a warm muslin cloth or flannel, wipe away the oil, taking the makeup with it. Simple!

 TOP TIP

Coconut oil is 'lipophilic', meaning it likes blending with other oils and thus breaks them down, making it a great makeup remover.

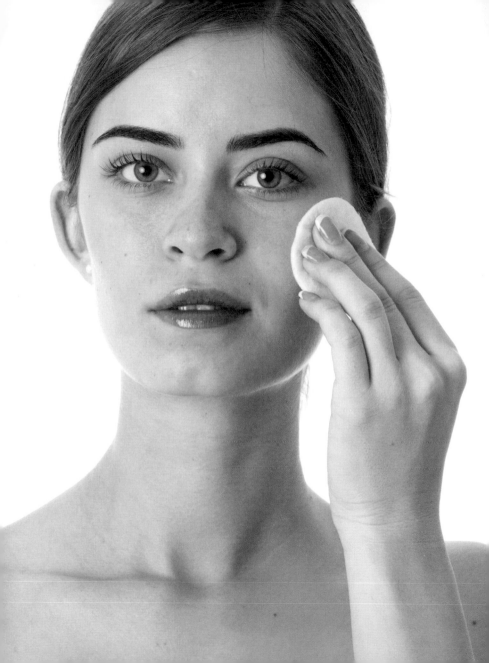

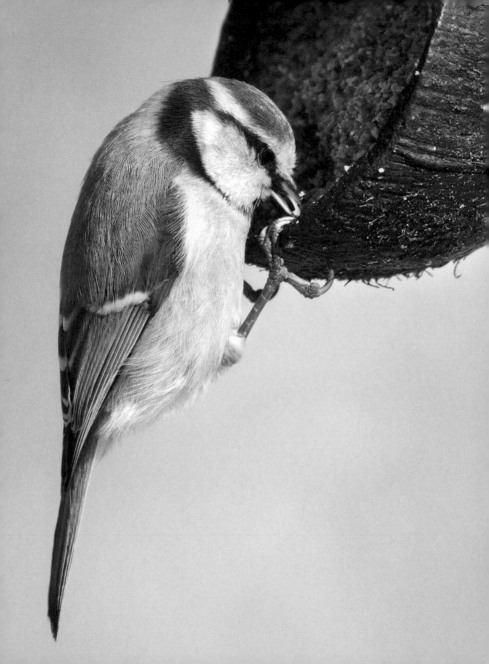

COCONUT BIRDFEEDER

Coconut shells make excellent sturdy birdfeeders and can be filled with nuts, lard or suet mixes to attract garden birds and keep them well fed all year round. Here's how to make a birdfeeder.

METHOD

First drill a hole in a whole coconut and drain out the milk.

After this you can simply cut the coconut in half along the longer side, using a hacksaw, then drill a hole to attach some twine, and fill with a suet or lard mixture that will cling to the shell when hung up. Find a nice spot in the garden and watch the birds enjoying their treat.

For a different version, after draining the coconut, cut it half-way through from the side, then half-way though from the top to meet the first cut and remove a quarter chunk of the shell.

This will create a hollow feeder with a little roof, Now drill a hole in the top. Add the garden twine to hang it up and fill with your favourite bird food mix.

💡 TOP TIP

Be very careful to ensure the coconut is secure while you are cutting, so it does not slip.

GROW YOUR OWN

Although you won't be self-sufficient in coconuts any time soon, it is possible to grow your own coconut tree and it makes an attractive container plant. Coconut trees grown in a pot will last around five years, as they rarely grow beyond the seedling stage in these conditions.

Choose a fresh coconut which still contains water (shake it to find out), and soak it in water for a couple of days. Place the soaked coconut with the point facing downwards in a large pot filled with moist peat compost, with a little sand or vermiculite added for optimum drainage. Leave around a third of the coconut above the soil.
The pot should be about 30cm deep to allow room for the roots to develop, although they have shallow roots so should not initially need a huge pot.

Keep the pot in a warm place, out of direct sunlight but ideally above 21°C, and water the soil well, without overwatering. If you do repot your tree, add more sand or vermiculite to keep the drainage effective.

It will take around three to six months for a sharp green shoot to appear and roots to form. You need to water the developing tree frequently and feed it with a good quality fertilizer. Keep it warm and out of draughts – remember, this is a tropical plant. After five or so years a trunk will form and after that the first fruits might appear if you are very lucky!

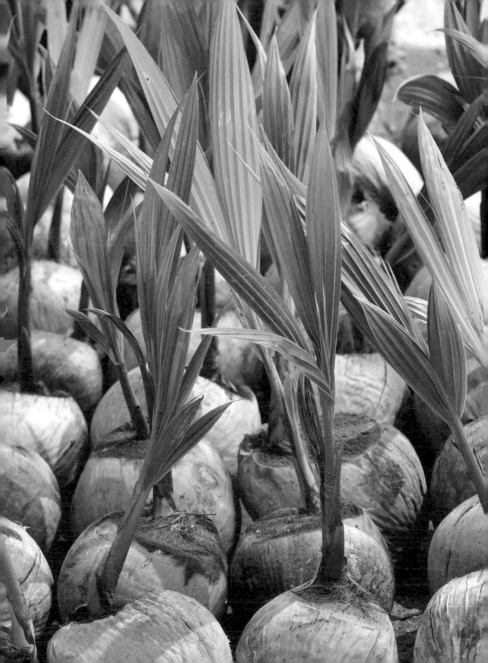

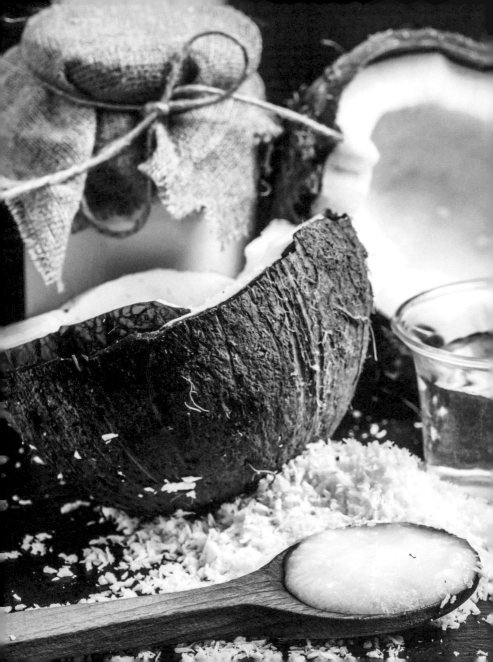

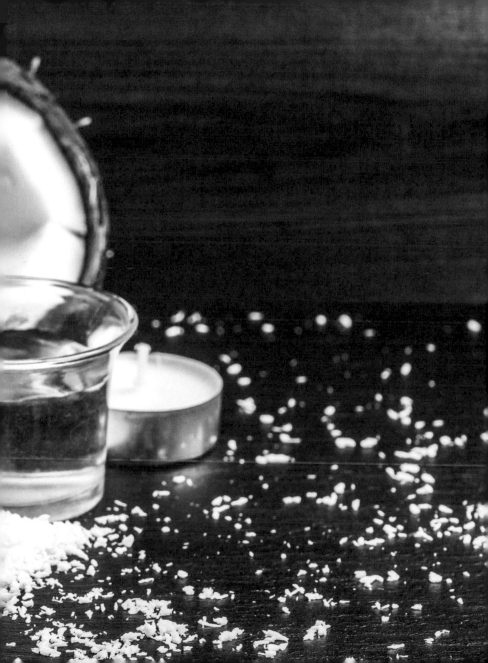

CONVERSION CHART
FOR COMMON MEASUREMENTS

LIQUIDS

15 ml	½ fl oz
25 ml	1 fl oz
50 ml	2 fl oz
75 ml	3 fl oz
100 ml	3 ½ fl oz
125 ml	4 fl oz
150 ml	¼ pint
175 ml	6 fl oz
200 ml	7 fl oz
250 ml	8 fl oz
275 ml	9 fl oz
300 ml	½ pint
325 ml	11 fl oz
350 ml	12 fl oz
375 ml	13 fl oz
400 ml	14 fl oz
450 ml	¾ pint
475 ml	16 fl oz
500 ml	17 fl oz
575 ml	18 fl oz
600 ml	1 pint
750 ml	1 ¼ pints
900 ml	1 ½ pints
1 litre	1 ¾ pints
1.2 litres	2 pints
1.5 litres	2 ½ pints
1.8 litres	3 pints
2 litres	3 ½ pints
2.5 litres	4 pints
3.6 litres	6 pints

WEIGHTS

5 g	¼ oz
15 g	½ oz
20 g	¾ oz
25 g	1 oz
50 g	2 oz
75 g	3 oz
125 g	4 oz
150 g	5 oz
175 g	6 oz
200 g	7 oz
250 g	8 oz
275 g	9 oz
300 g	10 oz
325 g	11 oz
375 g	12 oz
400 g	13 oz
425 g	14 oz
475 g	15 oz
500 g	1 lb
625 g	1 ¼ lb
750 g	1 ½ lb
875 g	1 ¾ lb
1 kg	2 lb
1.25 kg	2 ½ lb
1.5 kg	3 lb
1.75 kg	3 ½ lb
2 kg	4 lb

OVEN TEMPERATURES

110°C .... (225°F) .... gas mark ¼
120°C .... (250°F) .... gas mark ½
140°C .... (275°F) .... gas mark 1
150°C .... (300°F) .... gas mark 2
160°C .... (325°F) .... gas mark 3
180°C .... (350°F) .... gas mark 4
190°C .... (375°F) .... gas mark 5
200°C ..... (400°F) .... gas mark 6
220°C ...... (425°F) .... gas mark 7
230°C ...... (450°F) .... gas mark 8

MEASUREMENTS

5 mm .... ¼ inch
1 cm .... ½ inch
1.5 cm .... ¾ inch
2.5 cm .... 1 inch
5 cm .... 2 inches
7 cm .... 3 inches
10 cm .... 4 inches
12 cm .... 5 inches
15 cm .... 6 inches
18 cm .... 7 inches
20 cm .... 8 inches
23 cm .... 9 inches
25 cm .... 10 inches
28 cm .... 11 inches
30 cm .... 12 inches
33 cm .... 13 inches

KEY TO SYMBOLS

 Dairy free

 Gluten free

 Vegetarian

 Vegan

A NOTE ON USING DIFFERENT OVENS

Not all ovens are the same, and the more cooking you do the better you will get to know yours. If a recipe says that you need to bake something for ten minutes or until golden brown, use your judgment as to whether it needs a few extra minutes. Conversely don't overcook food by following the timings rigidly if you think it looks ready.

As a general rule gas ovens have more uneven heat distribution so the top of the oven may be hotter than the bottom. Electric ovens tend to maintain a regular temperature throughout and distribute heat more evenly, especially fan ovens.

All the recipes in this book have been tested in an electric oven with a fan. Recommended oven temperatures are provided for electric (Celsius and Fahrenheit), and gas. If you have a fan oven then lower the electric temperature by 20°.

Bloomsbury Publishing
An imprint of Bloomsbury Publishing plc

50 Bedford Square
London
WC1B 3DP
UK

1385 Broadway
New York
NY 10018
USA

www.bloomsbury.com

BLOOMSBURY and the Diana logo are trademarks of Bloomsbury Publishing Plc

First Published in 2017

© Bloomsbury Publishing plc

Created for Bloomsbury by Plum5 Ltd

Photographs and Illustrations © Shutterstock

British Library Cataloguing-in-Publication Data
A catalogue record for this book is available from the British Library.

Library of Congress Cataloguing-in-Publication Data
A catalogue record for this book is available from the Library of Congress.

ISBN: 9781408887202

2 4 6 8 10 9 7 5 3 1

Printed in China by C&C Printing

To find out more about our authors and books visit www.bloomsbury.com.
Here you will find extracts, author interviews, details of forthcoming events
and the option to sign up for our newsletters.